SUPERHERO
SIX-PACK
WITH CALISTHENICS

THE BODYWEIGHT TRAINING PROGRAM TO RIPPED ABS AND A POWERFUL CORE

MARKUS A. KASSEL

Table of Contents

Introduction: Abs Make the (Super)Man

It's kind of funny when you think about it. Abs represent such a small part of our body... Yet, entire careers have been built around them. I'm not saying it's the most solid foundation to base your future on, but where would Mark Wahlberg (aka Marky Mark) be today if his midsection had looked like he was going to hibernate for the next six months rather than the shredded six-pack that landed him his Calvin Klein stunt? You really think he sold discs and got involved in movies at first because of his artistic talents? **Plenty of actors and celebrities would still be pushing carts at Walmart if it wasn't for their flawless physique**.

I know, I'm not teaching you anything new... But some people would have you believe that this is a vain pursuit, that we shouldn't bother because what really counts is what's on the inside. To these fine ladies and gentlemen, I would simply say this: "C'MON! WAKE UP!"

Let's be realistic here for a second. Let's stop kidding ourselves, pretend like we're above all this and mistake a lack of willpower for intellectual superiority! Getting washboard abs is as worthy a goal as say learning a new language. Period! It's a challenge that will test your willpower and there's no shame in admitting it sits atop your to-do list! Just like with A.A., the first step is acceptance:

"Hello, my name is John and I'm a six-packoholic!"

One can be beautiful on the inside AND the outside! Have brains AND brawn!

However, if you've been struggling with your weight your entire life, if you forgot what your feet looked like because when you stare down all you see is your belly, it may seem like a faraway dream. A destination so distant that it sounds almost impossible to reach; like winning the lottery or getting a date with Penelope Cruz. You're ready to play the game but, deep inside, you don't think you stand a chance.

<u>That is about to change</u>!

In this book, **I will show you the step-by-step to losing the gut and getting the abs you've always wanted**. No matter your starting point, you too can lean down and secure the shredded look that only seems feasible if you live in Hollywood.

But that's not all! I will also show you the best exercises to strengthen your core and dramatically improve your health and athletic performances! If you still needed an excuse to start because you still subscribed to the "inside beauty" crap, there you go! You can feel relieved now. Training your abs will not only make you look like a stud; it will also **greatly enhance your quality of life**.

But what do I know anyway? Why should you listen to anything I have to say?

As I explained at length in my previous books, I was involved in a car accident when I was a teenager. I got run over as I was crossing the street and suffered multiple fractures and a concussion. It took me almost a whole year to recover and, during that time, I inflated like I was injecting my stomach full of synthol, which really messed with my self-confidence. At a time where we care a bit too much what our peers think of us, I was stuck with a good 30 pounds in excess. You can imagine how down and depressed I felt... But I never lost faith. I knew that even though the road ahead might be long, it was only a matter of time before I got to the end of it, IF I kept ploughing on.

And indeed, with much effort, trial and error, I eventually managed to lose most of that weight. I never reached the point where my abs were popping out or I could go shirtless without feeling a bit self-conscious, though. The truth is that I didn't really know what I was doing. **I succeeded despite my many mistakes**, by sheer persistence. Now, that's one way to go about it and slim down, but it sure ain't the fastest or the most fun, is it?

To make matters worse, I wasn't paying my core its due respect. I thought that, because I was already working out and fitting in a few crunches here and there, I didn't need to target it more specifically. To be completely honest, though it sounds stupid in retrospect, I thought my abdominals were in pretty good condition.

After all, with all the martial arts and bodyweight training I had done during my youth, how could it have been otherwise? I was bulletproof, right? Yeah, RIGHT!

Reality struck when I decided to try my hand at some Parkour. Young naive me registered for a free session and went with confidence, convinced that he would tear it up, American Ninja Warrior style... What I ended up tearing, though, wasn't the s*** but my lower abdominals!

After we warmed up, prepped our joints and got ready to start, the coach set up a few workshops to practice some basic acrobatics.

I walked towards the front flip group. The move seemed easy enough: jump on the trampoline, tuck the knees, turn on yourself and land on the mat. Piece of cake!

On my first attempt, as I launched into the air and tried to bring my knees to my chest, I felt a sharp pain rise in my right side. It turned out that I had strained it! So much for the powerful abs! I got sidelined for two weeks and couldn't move or train without wincing.

This taught me a valuable lesson: my abs were weaker than a pinky finger and I couldn't afford to neglect them anymore if I wanted to become as strong as I aimed to be. And so I started on another one of those quests that truly changed my life. I started experimenting, testing and refining core training techniques. When they didn't work, I ditched them; when they provided results, I tweaked them.

Pretty soon, **I saw an entire new world open to me**. As my understanding of good nutrition also improved, my abs began to come out of their hiding. But, more importantly, I started experiencing a lot of great side-effects. You see, training your core is essential to reaching your full physical potential and becoming a true life superhero.

If you've read any of my previous books, you know I'm all about functionality. In fact, that's what drove me to write the Real Life Superman series in the first place. To give you the most effective and actionable tips to not only pack on muscle and get stronger, but also to make you faster and more agile. To give you abilities that would serve you in your daily life and not just to show off at the beach.

I brought the same spirit to this guide. Here, I will share with you all I learned about getting the fat to disappear and forging powerful abs that will impact every other area of your life. You'll come to see that, in the end, aesthetics and functionality are but two sides of the same coin.

Why Developing a Strong Core Is a Must

Let's talk physics for a few seconds now, shall we? Don't worry, I'm not going to go all Friedmann on you and start dropping scary equations that'll give you nightmares for days. I just want to talk about breaking points.

Answer me this: usually, where is any object at its weakest? When you bend a piece of wood and continue to increase the force gradually, what happens?

Any body is almost always at its weakest at the center... and the human body is no exception! If it's frail at the middle, it will break like a twig when put under stress. As the saying goes, a chain is only as strong as its weakest link. The core is the hinge of the body; it requires extra care and attention to ensure it keeps the entire chain strong, stable and healthy.

Working the core is an absolute prerequisite to achieving any of the more advanced bodyweight movements... but you don't need to be involved with calisthenics to reap the rewards of specific abs training.

In fact, **strengthening the abdominals has been shown to increase your performance in any field**, whatever your hobbies or occupation. It can make you quicker or have you hit (with your fist or your foot) much harder.

How? Well, to return to the body-chain image we talked about, your core is the main link connecting the two extremities of your body which are your legs and your trunk. When you accomplish any task, from kicking a football to carrying a heavy bag, your abs will always get solicited at one point or another. Either directly, when the movement originates from your center, or indirectly as the force you've generated in your legs travels through your core to reach your hands (or vice versa.) Like when you're throwing a fastball.

At the very least, your core will play a stabilizing role and avoid power leakage. In short, your abs are the basis and support from which any movement gains momentum. **Keep them in poor condition and suffer the consequences**!

If that wasn't reason enough for you to start a core strengthening program, consider these other benefits:

- **Working your core will give you superior balance**: by helping to stabilize your torso and limbs, stronger abs will increase your balance and also make you move and change directions much quicker (perfect for football players and other athletes who need to catch their opponents off balance);
- **Working your core will improve your breathing**: specific core training will also reinforce your diaphragm which is critical to the breathing process. It will make every one of your inspirations much more deeper and effective. Thanks to a better oxygenation of your muscles and your brain, you will feel less stressed and more alert;
- **Working your core will boost your digestion**: feeling a bit bloated or constipated lately? Train the abs! With the exercises we'll see below, you will not only toughen up but lengthen your abdominals which, if they're too short or stiff, can squeeze your internal organs and prevent proper food assimilation;
- **Working your core will enhance your posture**: pretty self-explanatory. Since your abs help stabilize your back, improving their power and flexibility will go a long way towards acquiring the perfect posture;
- **Working your core will prevent back pain and limit injuries**: a corollary to the previous point, better abs will also mean less risk of developing back ache as

you'll be standing straighter and your spine will get more support. For the same reason, you'll benefit from extra protection against any shock, torsion or pressure you could sustain and that could result in an injury;

- **Working your core will make your bones much stronger**: last but not least, much like with bodyweight training, by targeting your abs and placing your bones under stress, you will make them stronger over time as the added pressure of the exercises will in turn increase their density.

As you can see, a lot of sweet benefits anyone looking to perform at his best would be foolish not to take advantage of!

But it's easier said than done, right? Can you just lie down, do a couple sit-ups, and expect to look like Gerard Butler in the 300's when you get up? You wish!

What's for sure is that **with all the crap we hear or read about in magazines**, not to mention those late-night infomercials that never seem to run out of "miracle" products that sell for a premium and that promise to get you ripped while you sleep, **it can get near impossible for the beginner to sort between truth and BS**. To know exactly what to do and avoid like the plague.

In short, to trust in a program that'll bring the desired results.

Don't worry buddy, Markus is here to set the record straight! Like I did with my Real Life Superman series where I showed you my tried and true method to become more muscular and develop your mental fortitude, I will teach you the quickest and most effective way to turn your jelly belly into a real piece of art, beautiful and extremely powerful!

You will learn how you too can **turn this weakness of yours into one of your main strengths**. So, if you're ready, buckle up and let's claim that superhero six-pack you've been waiting for!

Anatomy of a Six-Pack

Before we jump right into the program per se, we need to make the presentations. No, not with me, dude! You already know my old mug! I'm talking about your very own belly and soon-to-be object of beauty.

The best way to turn an enemy into a friend is to **get to know him intimately**. Learn how he functions and what makes him tick; that's how you'll win him over.

Know Thy Enemy

Yes, if we want to master our core, we first need to understand how it works. Don't panic, I won't be long. I promise it'll be over before your eyelids got to close completely shut, alright?

If you ever wondered where "abdominals" came from, it derives from the Latin word *abdomen* which in turn stems from *abdo*... that means "hidden." How funny, considering their origin, that we're actually fighting to get those suckers to show, huh?

You know, it's no coincidence that the abs take an "s" and are almost never used in their singular form. After all, the abdominals are not made up of one but an entire group of muscles; a **complex muscular network** where every unit will get involved, at a different level and intensity, depending on the motion in question. Got it?

According to your position, sitting or standing, lying on your side or on your back, it's not the same abs that will provide much of the work when you move.

And with that out of the way, let's take a closer look at the badboys:

- **Obliques**: they're located on your sides and comprise both the internal and external obliques. As their name would suggest, the external obliques cover the internal which are therefore invisible (duh!) They all originate from the ribs and attach themselves to the hip. They're the ones to give a shout out to whenever you want to turn at the waist or bend to the side;
- **Rectus Abdominis**: let's keep with the Latin here for a second, I know you love it... The *rectus abdominis* is THE 6-pack we generally refer to when we talk about the abs. It's a flat muscle that is quite large and which covers the entire front of your belly (from your breastbone to your willy – if you got one.) Any time you raise your knees, get up from bed or shorten the distance between your lower and upper body, it's the *rectus* which accomplishes the miracle;
- **Transversus Abdominis**: this one wraps around the stomach much like a weightlifting belt. But no matter how hard you work it, you'll never get to see its curves as that muscle is buried deep in the recesses of the abs. So, why train it at all? Like I said, this program is not only about looking good but performing to our best as well, and the *transversus* will help in that

sense. Not only is it involved in the breathing process, it also helps stabilize the spine and keep our guts nicely packed;

- **Erector Spinae**: I know, that one's located in the back, so why am I mentioning it here? Well, considering that it's part of the abdominal belt (as the lumbar muscles), it deserves a spot on this list. To be completely precise, it doesn't stop at the lower back but runs almost the entire length of it. We only get to see the bottom part because, at the top, it's drowned in the volume of bigger muscles such as the lats. The *erector spinae* is essential to extensions of the spine. That's the set of muscles that allow us to get back up when we fall, so we had better make them strong... if you see what I mean (wink, wink)!

In short, we'll want to work the *rectus abdominis* – of course! – as that's **what will grant us our most coveted 6-pack**... but we'll also beware of paying careful attention to the other muscles that make up the abdominals.

Failure to do so would only lead to imbalances down the road, weakness and drop in our performances.

Let's make it right from the start and cover all bases. You'll thank me later.

From 6 to 8-Pack?

While we're on the topic of anatomical details; I hear a lot of people asking how to go about securing an 8-pack, like it's the next natural step in developing your abs, like Goku aiming for SSJ2 after he managed to turn into the first Super Saiyan form.

And that reasoning is not without merits; it makes sense. By pushing your abs to their limits, you force them to grow and mature. It would only seem logical, after you've worked your butt off for months, that new muscle would start to show.

Unfortunately, the human body doesn't work that way. The shape – as well as the number – of your abs is predetermined; it's 100% genetics. You could quit your job and retreat into some lost cabin in the woods to do nothing but smash your abs, Shaolin style, for the next 10 years, their number would remain unchanged.

All you can do is make them stronger and bigger. That's quite something!

The REAL Secret behind Killers Abs
Alright, this is the bit you've been waiting for. This is where I reveal the foolproof method for leaning down and achieving a superhero six-pack.

So, open your eyes, keep them peeled and don't blink!

It's All about Fat
If you've ever set foot inside a gym, you've probably been witness to this scene: a guy killing himself day after day, performing hundreds and hundreds of crunches, as if he was trying to punish himself for some horrendous sin he couldn't bring himself to confess.

And despite his efforts, despite the sweat, the pain and the passing months, that guy remains exactly the same!

Is that person cursed? Are some poor devils destined to remain "heavy" because of their natural constitution?

Hell no!

There's no need to light candles to release any evil spell. The truth is that **most people simply go at the process completely wrong**. It's not always the will or the motivation that is lacking; it's often the knowledge. People just don't know what they're doing! We've been led to believe that, to lose the gut, we need to hit it harder than terrorist groups. But that couldn't be further from the truth.

One CANNOT lose weight from the belly simply by exercising it.

I know, that seems counterintuitive, but you can't choose where to thin down by targeting a specific area. This "spot reduction" myth is one of the most pervasive in the field and, every day, thousands of poor shmucks fall victim to it.

Of course, you burn calories when you bust your butt off with sit-ups... but in the same manner that chewing gum will never hollow your cheeks, don't count on those movements to create the stomach of an Adonis. Training the abs with the exercises recommended by most coaches doesn't burn that many calories anyway.

So, what to do?

The big secret to protruding abs is to reach a certain level of body fat. Simple as that. You could be the lucky owner of the most beautiful 6-pack on planet Earth, if you're above the limit, you'll never know it! On the other hand, if you're concentration camp thin but got no muscle to your abs, we won't see a thing either but your bones.

Thus, we'll need to ensure you attain the right percentage WITH the right stuff under your shirt!

Before we proceed with our plan of attack, let's see how to measure your own levels, so we know what we're facing and exactly how much work we got ahead of us, OK?

How to Measure Your Body Fat Percentage

There's at least half a dozen ways to calculate that percentage, with varying prices and scores of reliability.

The number one option, without a doubt, has to be the DXA (for Dual Energy X-Ray Absorptiometry.) Sounds like a new secret weapon in development by DARPA, right? By making use of densitometry, this method allows a precise calculation of your bones, muscles and fat %, to one decimal place.

Here's how we're going to get our percentage then, right?

Erm, how to say this... Unless you got a Benjamin to waste on this exam, we'll have to pass as the prohibitive cost isn't justified. We'll also have to forget about using the BMI, as is often recommended by doctors. Why? Because the results would be skewed; this formula doesn't work for people with a muscle mass that's over the average.

OK but, if we can't use those, what techniques have we left to achieve our goal?

- **Get out the measuring tape**: here, you will get your body fat percentage by utilizing a complex equation involving your weight, age, as well as the measures from your hips, neck, waist... If you'd like to try that method, make it easier on you and use an online calculator. But frankly, I'm not a big fan of it because, once again, the results might be skewed depending on your specific morphology (huge neck, thin waist, large hips...);
- **Get yourself some calipers**: want to get your numbers but don't feel like breaking the bank? For the price of a Big Mac meal, you can purchase a pair of calipers that will get the job done. Simply follow the guidelines that you'll find with the device and take measures at specific points like the back, the arms... The reliability is only to a few percent, but that should give you a rough estimate of where you're standing, for cheap;
- **Hop on biometric scales**: also known as "body fat" or "bioelectric impedance" scales, these work just like your regular scales; they can tell how much you weigh when you step on them. But, more valuable to us here, they can analyze your body composition by sending a current through your body that will give out the percentage of each tissue. Although some people only swear by them, I'm frankly not impressed. I find they're too flaky in their readings because their

precision can fluctuate depending on the volume of water you're holding, for example.

In the end, don't go pulling your hair. Order some calipers on the Net and take a few minutes to take the measurements. It may not be the very best option but, like I said, calipers are cheap and we don't need to know your body fat percentage down to the last decimal point anyway.

Now you've got your digits; it's time to assess the damage!

From Steven Seagal to the Incredible Hulk

Numbers don't lie. So, let's man up and see where we're standing.

You're over 26% body fat: sorry to break the news but you've been going a bit too heavy on the snacks, my friend! It's time to roll up your sleeves and get to work! For now, forget all about getting a six-pack... I don't want to sound like a wet blanket or lecture you but we're talking about your health here. Your first target will be to go below 20% to reduce cardiovascular and other associated risks.

You're between 25-18% body fat: at this stage, you've not yet lost sight of your toes but that shouldn't be long if you continue to pack on the pounds. Your abs are still nowhere to be seen.

You're between 17-14% body fat: OK, we're slowly getting there. You don't need much for your six-pack to start to show. This is the level of body fat of people who're said to be "in shape."

You're between 12-7% body fat: great, you're already quite on the ripped side! Whatever it is you're doing, continue to do it because it seems to be working. I would only suggest you implement the exercises we'll see below to further strengthen your core. This is the range most people are targeting when they're looking to get a six-pack. We'll aim for 10%, as far as we're concerned. You'll look great at that number and you'll be able to keep it without too much hassle.

You're below 6% body fat: damn, dude! Put some clothes on your back; you're going to catch a cold! This is how lean professional bodybuilders can get for a contest. It's not advised to keep such low numbers for any length of time as your body needs a certain level of body fat to function optimally. That's why getting so low won't be any of our business here.

If all this talk still doesn't ring a bell and you'd rather have a visual aid, here's a chart to show you what each category looks like. As the saying goes: a picture is worth a thousand words, right?

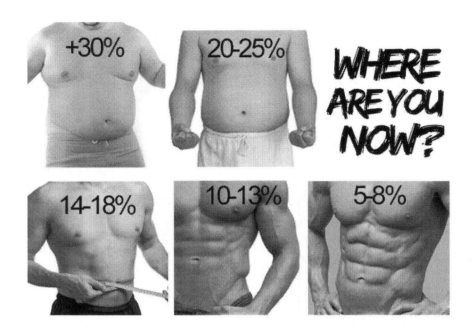

PS: small aside; although my guides are primarily targeted towards men, if you're a girl and you're reading this, you can still refer to the numbers we just stated above. Just add 7% to any "category" to account for a naturally higher percentage of fat with women.

The Magic Formula

If, like we've discovered much to our dismay, driving ourselves silly with abs exercises will not be enough to force our abs out, **we'll have to combine our core training with other techniques to get that body fat down**.

Ultimately, the program we're going to put into place will not only include specific routines to develop your abdominal power and allow you to perform impressive feats of strength, but also nutrition guidelines and a few cardio exercises.

Without going into too much detail, to succeed in that sense, we'll have to burn more calories than we're taking in. It's really no rocket science; it's a simple addition-subtraction operation.

And to get there, we've got several options – from training with high intensity to applying low carb or intermittent fasting concepts. But in the end, whichever road you decide to embark on, the general formula will remain identical:

Abs Training + Diet + Cardio = Superhero Six-Pack

Tools of the Trade – What You'll Need

OK, now we've got a better understanding of what awaits us. You're still motivated to follow through? Attaboy!

First things first, let's discuss the equipment we'll need to bring our abdominals up to par.

Gym or Gymless?

For those of you who like to keep an eye on the fitness industry, you've probably already noticed that, every week, it seems like some company has just made the revolutionary breakthrough that will forever change the face of the Earth.

Every week, there's a new miracle device that hits the market and which promises to get you from blob to Terminator in only 5 minutes per day!

It doesn't matter that a thousand other products made similar claims in the past with dubious results; this time, it's for real! It has to be! Look at the shape of the guy in the ad. He sure seems to know what he's doing. So, that machine has to work, right? Yes, this time, thanks to this baby, your wish will be granted: you'll get a sexy stomach without breaking a sweat or even getting winded. You know what? You'll even get to eat potato chips while you're at it!

The big joke!

Miracle abs devices are like Santa. At one point, even though it's hard, you've got to admit they don't exist.

To tell you the truth, I'd go as far as saying that you don't even need a machine or weights to train your abs. As long as you've got a floor to lie down on, you should be good to go. You can invest in a rubber floor mat for a few bucks if you want, to protect your back. And a pull-up bar, as we'll need something to hang from for the more advanced variations of our moves... But, like I said, nothing is compulsory.

That's why, if you don't have a gym membership yet, I won't have you cough up the money. Now, I'm not saying that gyms are completely worthless as they do have their use. For example, they can be good to keep you accountable in the beginning as you'll want to get your money's worth, every month. It would suck big time to have them take our hard-earned dough and not benefit, wouldn't it?

Also, going to a gym gives you access to barbells to work on your squats and other beneficial lifts... but, at the risk of repeating myself, it's absolutely not needed to accomplish our mission here. Your own bodyweight will suffice.

In fact, training with your bodyweight instead of free weights or machines is the superior option on a lot of levels...

The Many Advantages of Bodyweight Training

When you see all the beefcakes who've made the gym their home, it may seem stupid not to rush there as well if you want to look a quarter like them. Why change a winning recipe?

Before I answer this, let's go back to our goals for one second. What are we trying to achieve with this program?

First, we're looking to lose weight so that our abs become noticeable. Two, we want to turn them into an indestructible armor while keeping our speed and explosiveness intact. In other words, we're not really trying to end up looking like the Mountain in GoT... not that there's anything wrong with that, but we're rather aiming for an athletic physique. We want to look ripped, sharp and muscular – yes – but not overly so. In short, we want to strike the perfect balance between all those attributes.

And for THAT type of objectives, bodyweight training just has no rival.

Here are some of its main benefits:

- Completely free;
- Not limited by time or place;
- Natural movements (vs mechanical);
- Explosive;
- Gradual;
- Works the balance;
- Fun and challenging;
- Prepares the joints = injury prevention;
- Comprehensive;
- …

You might be reading this list and go: "OK, I can figure how it would work in the beginning to strengthen my abs… but how can my sole bodyweight provide enough stimulation in the long run to keep my abs on edge and force them to grow?" In other words, is this method effective even for more experienced athletes?

Well, allow me to introduce you to a neat principle that's called "**tweaking the mechanical advantage**": as we gain strength, and the exercises become too easy for us to still gain (muscle and strength), we will modify them in such a manner as to decrease our leverage.

We'll make those movements harder and harder by changing the position of our limbs and trunk so that our muscles are now at their weakest.

Take the example of a simple plank: you're in a push-up position and you can hold the movement for quite some time. What happens now if you move your head forward (while keeping your arms locked) so that your shoulders are a few inches <u>in front</u> of your hands instead of right above? Yes, there will be extra pressure/torque on your pecs, shoulders and abdominals, and it'll be harder to hold the position the further away you stray from the vertical.

By changing the angle at which the strength is applied, you put yourself at a greater mechanical disadvantage.

Capisce?

Our training program will make full use of that principle. We'll be starting every exercise with an easy variation and progress towards positions where our abs will get the crap beaten out of them.

Solving the Diet Puzzle

Alright, we've seen thus far that our program will have 2 main objectives:

- **Keeping you in a caloric deficit** so that your levels of fat decrease and your abdominal muscles get a chance to shine;
- **Building an insanely strong core** that will enhance your performance on all levels, preserve your health and make you look like a stud.

When it's presented that way, it seems so simple... Yet, it took me years to understand that I had to focus on both evenly if I was to achieve the results I was hoping for. It's only when I did this that my six-pack started to pop out.

And the first item we need to take care of is your diet. Even more so than cardio and core training – which represent the other two pillars of this program –, a clean and healthy diet is an absolute prerequisite to killer abs. You HAVE TO get your eating under control. Unless your name is Dean Karnazes and you burn through 10,000 calories on some days (and can therefore indulge a little), you will need to be strict.

In the following pages, we will see 3 different ways to go about tweaking our diet.

I'll detail each one of them, with their pros and cons, and give you my personal take at the end. I prefer to give you some options because I understand that not everybody may feel ready to totally revamp the way they're eating.

The Regular Approach

This is the type of diet you usually find in your average fitness magazine and, if you've been interested in dieting for any length of time, it's probably the technique you already tried.

Although it has taken a lot of different names throughout the years, to make it more "marketable" and keep people flashing their wallet, the reasoning behind this approach remains the same: **eating less calories than we use**.

Just like with Weight Watchers and their points system, the main focus will be on ensuring the body is "underfed" and has no choice but to go and dig into our fat reserves to fuel its daily needs.

Which means that, before we even learn how to tweak the way we eat, we first need to find our daily energy requirements.

How to Calculate Your Daily Caloric Needs

Lots of formulas have been invented to find that number... but the most reliable has to be the Sterling-Pasmore equation which starts with finding out your basal metabolism (i.e. the energy required for your body to fulfill its vital functions):

Energy required at rest = lean mass x 13.8kcals

To find your lean mass, simply subtract your pounds of fat from your overall weight. Say you're a 180lbs guy and you're at 20% BF, your lean mass will be: 180 - (180x20%) = 144lbs

Once you got that number, you'll have to multiply it by a factor that will account for your level of activity throughout the day. Of course, your caloric needs won't be the same whether you spend your days as a bed tester or you're fishing king crab in Alaska.

- For people who stay seated behind a desk most of the day, this factor will be equal to 1.2
- If you're training at a low intensity or move around a bit, make it 1.375
- If that training is more thorough and you work out 3 to 5 times a week, multiply by 1.55
- Once you're exercising at a high intensity (or working a very labor intensive job) pretty much every day, you'll need 1.725 times your basal metabolic rate
- Last but not least, we've got the 1.9 factor... but, unless you're getting ready for the Olympics or mining coal from dusk to dawn, forget about it.

In our previous example, we looked at a 180lbs man with a bodyfat percentage approaching the 20%. Now, if that guy is quite active and working out 3 times a week, the number of calories he'll need to keep his weight stable is:

$$(180lbs - (180x20\%)) \times 13.8 \times 1.55 = 3080 \text{ kcals}$$

Thus, to start losing our gut, we'll have to shoot below that number. But by how much exactly?

For starters, experiment with a 400 decrease. Keep at it for a whole week before reevaluating. If you notice you're losing weight, continue. If you see no apparent results, take off 200 more, then 200 more... The goal here is to find the sweet spot where you're burning fat but you're not depriving yourself too much. Going overboard and reducing your calories too drastically would kill your performance (remember that we still need energy to work our core afterwards) and mess with your mood.

As you can figure out, that number can quickly dwindle to a point where you don't get to eat much from the day! That's one more reason to introduce cardio training to our program as it will allow us to bump our caloric intake a bit and still lose weight.

Pros, Cons & Considerations
If you decide to go with this approach, you need to **make sure you get enough protein** with your meals to repair muscle damage and guarantee your abs get everything they need to thrive.

Forget what your family physician said about eating one 4 ounces piece of meat a day! Bump your intake so that proteins represent 30% of your overall calories, with carbs and fats making the remaining 45% and 25%.

All in all, you should ingest close to 1g of protein per pound of bodyweight. If you're not used to eating that much meat/fish/eggs, it may be hard in the beginning... That's why I recommend you divide your meals up so that you don't eat 3 times a day but rather every 3 hours (or about 5/6 meals.) Eat less but more often.

Tips for Cutting Your Calories with Ease
Our target being to lower our calories without starving ourselves, every bit will help. The last thing we want is to feel famished; that's the surest way to fail. We want to **find a plan we can live with**, not one that would make our life miserable. If you struggle too much, you may be strong for a while... but there will eventually come a time when you end up throwing in the towel.

No one can be solid 24/7.

Including some of the following tips in your plan will greatly help in dropping your daily amount of calories while still ensuring you feel relatively satiated:

- **Before any meal, drink a tall glass of water**: simply put, water takes up space. By starting every meal with a few generous sips from your glass, you'll pre-fill your stomach;
- **Double your servings of veggies**: if meat is essential for building our abdominal muscles, veggies will be the actual key to losing the fat that surrounds them. Whatever vegetable is on the menu today, you can gorge without any remorse. You'll always be full

before you have a chance to do any damage to your waistline. Veggies are low on calories and chock-full of nutrients and vitamins. So, why limit them?

- **Use and abuse of spices**: eating a pound of steamed cooked greens can become old real quick if you use nothing but salt & pepper to give the bastards some taste. Enter spices! Instead of using sauces which are way too rich (and this goes for cooking meat too), pick some herbs and spices such as garlic, basilica, curry, pili-pili, curcuma and other delicious aromas which will keep your taste buds happy without any extra calories;
- **Favor fiber rich products**: the funny thing about fiber, and which is of interest to us, is that 1) we can't digest it, and 02) it takes a lot of room. Thus, eating foodstuff rich in fiber (like beans, cereals, almonds, figs) will slow down our digestion and make us feel full for a long time;
- **Skip the dessert**: that one's a no-brainer. If you want to cut your calories, avoid the Ben & Jerry's;
- **Drop the soda**: did you know that one glass of regular soda was about 100kcals? And the worst about it is that we can seldom just have one... Once you've opened the bottle, you've got to finish it, right? Drop that crap and your belly (and your heart and your kidneys and your liver and your brain) will be grateful;
- **Breathe in, relax, and take it easy**: relax, man. Take some time to breathe between two mouthfuls. This is neither a race nor a contest; you shouldn't be eating

like there's a nuclear bomb about to drop and you wanted to get a last bite before you bit the dust. Eat consciously. Be aware of what you're doing. Better yet, be completely absorbed. Don't do anything else when you're eating. Focus on the smell, the taste, the texture of the food. Take in the full experience. Most of the time, we're done eating and we don't even remember what we just put in our mouth. If you're going to get calories in, might as well savor them to the full!

Yes, no, maybe?

This method has worked for a lot of people and it has a few things going in its favor. For one, it allows you to keep eating pretty much the same food as today but with a few arrangements/concessions (there are no forbidden food categories.)

Also, for straightforward people who like things clear and precise, this approach is based on measurable data that they can then tweak and analyze (no guesswork.)

However, one of its main drawbacks is that **it can be a drag and take out a lot of your time**. Here, every food item must be weighed and each calorie accounted for. You must also ensure that you respect the ratio of nutrients. It's not the best choice for you if you hate keeping a log.

Another notch on the cons side is that, except if you up your veggies intake and really clean up your act, the effects on your health will be limited.

The Paleo Approach

OK, so you just read through the previous section and said to yourself "been there, done that"?

If you've already tried one of that diet's gazillion variations but never got it to work, here's another alternative that might succeed where all the others failed.

The paleo diet aims to have you eat like our forefathers who inhabited this planet millions of years before us. It is based around the principle that our physiology has barely changed since those days and that, therefore, our body is much more adapted to their way of eating than the regular American diet of today full of processed foods and products of the agriculture which only date back a few millennia.

And it makes sense when you think about it. Seeing how slow evolution is, it would be no wonder that **our body had no time yet to get used to grains** and other such foods that we've only recently introduced into our meals.

Thus, going paleo means to go back to a hunter-gatherer diet which is mainly composed of meat and pretty much anything you can find in the wild, such as tubers, vegetables, berries and nuts.

All Cals Are Created Equal... Not!

I will not go in depth about what's wrong with eating grains and dairy products (which are the two main food categories that are being left out of the paleo diet) because I already have in my previous books... but let's just say for the record that the gluten and lactose they hold are no joke. They can mess with your digestive system and lead to all kinds of unpleasantness to say the least such as allergies, bloating, infections, irritable bowel...

No matter how serious those conditions can be, the main beef the paleo diet has with regular diets is that they rely way too heavily on carbs. That is already bad enough under normal conditions, but it reveals to be a nightmare when trying to lose weight!

Why? Not only does eating sugar leads to eating more of the yummy stuff (you know the feeling, right? When you promised yourself you would only have one bite of that chocolate and you ended up devouring the entire bar, with a pack of cookies that was lying next to it for good measure)... When you take in carbs, your body will react with an insulin spike that **marks the start of a real snowball effect that will wreak havoc in your body**.

Following that sugar rush, like with any drug, you'll feel the coming down hit you hard. Apathy and a foggy mind are often part of the deal as are hunger pangs.

Ever wondered why you were always so ravenous, despite all the food you ate? Here might be the culprit! And it wouldn't be fun if that was it, now would it? That's why insulin is also the main responsible for storing extra energy as fat (i.e. high insulin levels amplify the transport of dietary fat into your adipose tissue! Yeeha!)

Thus, for paleo converts, you couldn't possibly reduce your diet to a simple calculation. Ingesting 2,000 calories worth of beef does NOT produce the same results as getting those calories from Twizzlers and Skittles.

All calories are not created equal. This also implies that, as long as it comes from a quality source, you'll be able to eat MORE of the product.

Paleo Pros and Cons

The biggest pro in favor of the paleo diet is that it gets you rid of the number one cause of failure with most diets, and that is sugar.

Once you take that poison off your system, you'll see how better you'll feel. Not only will the pounds melt away, you'll feel more energetic and alive than ever before. And you won't have to suffer those horrendous cravings that come with eating carbs.

Studies have shown that sticking to the paleo principles can reverse type-2 diabetes, greatly reduce the risks of cardiovascular disease and so on... but that's not the topic of this particular book. If all we care about is our waistline, it will still prove extremely useful.

By taking most sources of carbohydrates off your diet, you will – after some adaptation time – **turn from a carb to a fat burner**. What does that mean? Essentially, your body will re-learn how to use fat (from your meals and from that pile you've got sitting around the middle) as its main source of energy. Thus, you will burn fat more quickly and with much more efficiency.

Also, with the paleo diet, you won't have to count a single calorie. If you're the type that just hates to weigh everything, this is the perfect choice. No counting because there'll be no use for it; just eat when you're hungry. The foods you'll be taking in are so nutrient-rich that you'll always be full before you could absorb too many calories.

With that being said, the paleo diet is not all rosy. Like every plan that aims to restrict us, it has its downsides. For one, it WILL make you feel like crap at first as your body gets weaned off the carbs. That state, which is called "low carb flu", is not the most pleasurable to be in and it can last up to a few weeks before it subsides.

Another weakness of this diet is that it offers less food choice than most. And when I say "less", I mean like "heck, I can't even have my bread, my pasta and my cereals anymore" type of less.

Last but not least, **it can get pretty expensive** if you try and follow every guideline.

The Intermittent Fasting Approach
Another alternative to leaning down with ease and which is worth taking a look at is intermittent fasting or IF.

The logic is simple: you want to bring your overall calorie count down? Stop eating for a certain amount of time, a few times a week.

No food = no calories. Voilà! How easier could it be?

Usually, **fasting twice a week is sufficient to getting satisfying results**. Once you've had your last meal of the day, don't take any more solid food (liquids are okay, as long as you refrain from the obvious no-no's like Coke and beer) until the next evening.

As with the regular approach, start small and adapt depending on how your body reacts. No need to go overboard if two days are enough to get your weight down.

The Body in the Fasting State

Before you protest and start calling me names, as the description of this approach conjures up images of people who have gone on a hunger strike and ended up looking like Christian Bale in The Machinist, don't worry, you won't be losing your hard earned muscle.

Staying in this state can lead to muscle loss but ONLY if you overdo it and fast for long periods of time without giving your body some rest. That's why we'll keep our sessions apart and never fast for more than 16-24 hours.

What's great about IF is the other physiological changes it induces. The moment your body gets free of the burden of digestion (which takes up a lot of resources), it can now attend to other maintenance tasks it may not usually get enough time to perform. IF will thus promote cellular repair, clean up toxins, and fight off infection. Neat, isn't it?

To top it off, it offers the same benefits as calorie restriction – which has been shown, in lab tests, to significantly prolong life expectancy – without any of the side-effects. And it increases insulin sensitivity, provides stronger resistance to stress and clears up the mind. Yep, just that.

Intermittent Fasting Pros & Cons

On a pure "will it get me my 6-pack?" level, intermittent fasting strikes by its convenience. It's so easy to implement **you could literally start right away without needing any other form of introduction**! You won't get a headache calculating your macros or trying to figure out if you can eat this or that...

IF will speed up your metabolism as well, which will ensure that even more calories are burned during your fast.

On the cons side, we can note that hunger may pose a problem. If you can't stand the idea of having your stomach hurt because it's so empty, this might not suit you. Though it does get better with time and the hunger eventually fades away, it will take a strong will to begin with.

Also, this approach might not be advisable if you suffer from medical conditions such as diabetes.

Last but not least, fasting may give you a false sense of security and you might end up doing more harm than good. What I mean is that you may be tempted to think that, because you're not eating during a few hours, you've got a license to gorge once it's over. Remember that intermittent fasting is no miracle pill. For it to work, you first need to get your nutrition under control.

The "Right" Answer to the Puzzle

In case you hadn't noticed yet, I'm partial to the paleo diet. In my eyes, it's the perfect solution for people who want not only to get ripped but to be in the best health possible... I'm so categorical about it because I've truly tried all the other options, and this is the one that gave me the best results by far!

Like I said, though, it's only my personal experience. That's why you're free to experiment with the aforementioned approaches to note how your own body reacts, and see from there.

Intermittent fasting can be a tremendous ally in losing fat and kicking your metabolism into high gear, and you can use it on its own or combine it with any sort of diet.

As for counting your calories and taking a mathematical approach to slimming down, that's how most bodybuilders proceed to get in contest shape, so it sure provides results if you can stick to it.

In the end, know that the 3 options work; **they're all different means to reach the same end**. I would simply add, in closing, that IF and the paleo principles are truly a way of life... It's not about dieting for a certain amount of time (like you could be with a regular approach to losing weight); once you've integrated them into your routine, it's usually for the long haul! This can be scary, thinking that you may be leaving your old ways behind forever (like you're abandoning a little piece of yourself in the process), but this is the surest way to ensure you never regain those pounds you lost. This is the surest way to keep reaping those health benefits for the decades to come!

Burn through Calories like a Freight Train

Cardio training, you usually hate it or learn to live with it (or you must be some kind of masochistic psycho if you like it)! Picture yourself on the stationary bike, cycling away as if you were getting ready for the Tour de France... You're pushing and pushing; 15 minutes have passed and, your legs on fire, you look at the screen to find out you've burned the whole of 30kcals! Rings any bell?

I know, cardio sucks! But it's a necessary evil on the road to getting ripped as your diet will only get you so far. You need to get your calories down without cutting too much into your food intake.

Wait, don't run away! I was being overly dramatic to emphasize the point. There's no need to cry or be scared. The truth is that, contrary to most people's experience, **cardio training does NOT have to be a chore** you'd be happy to trade for a date with your dentist.

No, even though you may choose to run on a treadmill, use the elliptical, the rowing machine or the bike, you don't have to. Cardio can be fun! In essence, any activity can become a cardio session; it doesn't have to happen in a gym, with your butt locked indoors.

Say you like basketball, why not call up a few friends and go and shoot hoops? You like walking? Put on your trekking shoes and go for a few miles in the forest or the park! The bottom line is that you need to move to burn calories. It doesn't matter how. What does matter though is that, to make a habit out of it, it will always work better if you pick an activity you like/love.

Two Ways to Skin the Cardio Cat

As I implied, there's a gazillion ways to do cardio. But if we had to categorize them, we could argue that there are 2 main groups to which they can all be linked. And those categories represent two different ways to approach your training.

First of all, you can go at it with low to moderate intensity. That's where most activities belong and that's probably how you envision cardio when I utter the word; that is, long and continuous effort like jogging. And as I mentioned, if you like it that way, then by all means stick with it... But a lot of people get bored pretty fast because, let's be honest here, it's not the most exhilarating thing in the world! Slow and steady wins the race but, look at the turtle, is she having any fun?!

Worse, as the output remains low throughout, the number of calories burned per unit of time will follow the trend. Which brings us to another issue people have expressed towards this type of cardio: it requires hours per week to show any visible results. And, with their busy schedule, most folks don't have that amount of time to dedicate to it.

Enter the second way to perform cardio, which takes the complete opposite view: high intensity training.

High Intensity for Maximum Results

The first time I heard about high intensity training, I must admit I was kind of skeptical. I had been so brainwashed by the common wisdom – that has it that you must be ready to do cardio for hours on end to get any kind of result – that it seemed like BS to me. Lose fat with only a few minutes of work? And Halle Berry would be bringing you a fresh towel after that? Sounded like those miracle diet pills that always end up being a scam.

Anyway, that's what HIIT proposes: for only 10-15 minutes of your time, it will provide maximum calorie expenditure.

How is that possible? How can you get any result with such low time under pressure?

The principle is simple; you will alternate all-out effort with resting periods until the allotted time is up. Those periods of extreme intensity will have you burn calories as you perform the exercise... but, if that was it, then you'd be right in thinking that it can't get you to lose much fat.

Where high intensity work really outshines the competition is in its ability to have you **continue to burn calories hours AFTER you're done** and you're back home enjoying a well-earned rest. It will significantly ramp up your metabolism in what is known as the "afterburn effect"!

Thus, for a much shorter training time, you'll consume more calories overall. Also, the fact that you can't go at it half-assedly and need to give it your 100% makes it both fun and challenging. Try to get bored as you push your body to its limits... Not going to happen! High intensity sessions can therefore keep you motivated where other more leisurely activities would stop presenting any allure after a while.

By keeping the sessions brief and sweet, HIIT will also preserve muscle mass. I won't go into much detail here but I'll simply say this: compare the physique of sprinters (or CrossFitters, for that matter, as they also train with severe bursts of energy) with that of long-distance runners. On one hand, you have ripped and muscular guys who are also extremely explosive. On the other, you have fast guys with stamina who look like sticks.

No option is ultimately better than the other but, if you're looking to build a physique that sets you apart from the average Joe, I guess you'll be more likely to lean towards the first type, won't you be?

In short, **train little but train hard** and reap the rewards.

High Intensity Routines

If you insist on following a low intensity training routine, there's not much explaining that needs to be done. Schedule at least 1h at a time; start running, cycling or whatever, and bite the bullet until it's over. Good luck!

Some experts would recommend that you stay within 60% of your maximum heart rate, what they call the "fat burning zone", but I call BS on their claim... If you're not training at high intensity, your heart rate won't change much to how much fat you end up losing.

If, on the other hand, you want to give high intensity training a try, here's how to proceed. I'll take sprints to illustrate the concept as that's the most common form and the easiest to put into practice:

- Use an Olympic track if you got one nearby or simply find a flat road/path that's clear of any object/obstacle;
- Run for 100-150 meters as quickly as you can;
- Walk back to your starting point to catch your breath, and restart the cycle;
- Alternate between this sprinting and walking for 10 minutes;
- (Crawl back home if you still got enough strength or call an ambulance to come and pick you up, ha ha.)

As the training becomes easier, to keep the intensity high, you can either up the time to 15 minutes, increase your speed, reduce your recovery time by jogging back to your starting line, or change terrains for a steeper slope.

Yep, no rocket science either. **Go balls to the wall, rest, and go at it again. That's the essence of high intensity training**.

That principle can be applied to nearly any physical activity, like the other approach. Some drills that I like to use in my own program include:

- **Jumping rope**: if you got a rope lying around, you can get one heck of a good workout. Jump and bring your knees to your chest fast for about 20-30 seconds, then take about the same time to rest by jumping slowly (or stopping altogether if you're too tired) until you repeat the maneuver, again and again, till the 10 minutes are off;
- **Rowing**: same thing with this one, provided that you got access to a rowing machine. Row as quickly as possible for 20 seconds (or give yourself a distance to cover), catch your breath, rinse and repeat;
- **Bag work**: I like to mix things up and often put on my boxing gloves for some bag work high intensity training. I will punch the bag with all my speed and power for intervals of 15-20 seconds. It will have your arms beg for mercy;
- **Stairs**: got no equipment at hand and don't feel like doing sprints? Take it to the stairs and run up the flight again and again!
- **WOD type of routine**: another great way to approach HIIT is with basic calisthenics moves like burpees, tuck jumps, air squats, pushups and mountain climbers... Accomplish intervals of around 8-12 repetitions. Deadly effective.

How Many Sessions per Week?

How to strike the best balance between too little and too much as far as cardio training is concerned? HIIT can be taxing on the body if performed too often... You need to let your organism rest but, on the other hand, doing it only once a week won't burn enough calories to be worth your while.

As a rule of thumb, I like to go for 3 sessions – or once every other day – that you can execute at the same time as your abs training.

Now, is it better to start with the cardio portion or to wait until <u>after</u> you've worked out?

There are proponents of both methods, and I can understand where they're all coming from as, no matter which part you begin with, that's the one that'll get your best effort. The exercise you'll save for the end will get the least output as you'll be tired already.

It's for that very reason that some people would have you train cardio and muscles on separate days... but, like I said, that's not a good idea. If you have too much to do and it takes up too much of your free time, there's a higher risk you'll end up quitting altogether. We need something we can live with, and **3 workout sessions a week seems to be the sweet spot**; it ensures enough stimulation for growth while offering a frequency that can be maintained in the long run.

So, what are we going to start with? In my eyes, the most important part of our training will be the abs. We will need every bit of strength we can muster to graduate through the progressions; thus, I would recommend you do the cardio at the end of the session. Sure, you'll have less energy but, on the other hand, your glycogen stocks will already have been hit, which means you'll burn even more fat!

Extra Tips for Losing More Calories

In the battle against flab, **every little calorie we can manage to burn eventually adds up**; it's like those droplets that fall and fall, and don't seem to make any kind of difference... until the last one makes the cup run over!

In addition to our diet and cardio training sessions, there are a few habits we can take up that don't demand much efforts but that can weigh in the balance. All they require is that you get out of your lazy mood and make the decision to be more active in your everyday life.

Start doing the following and regain control over your waistline:

- **Walk**: it doesn't get easier than this; walk and watch the pounds slowly drop. This is the number one tip I would advise you include in your daily routine. Whether you choose to go to work on foot, to park a little further away to have a good 10 to 15 minutes of walking time, or to stop taking the car altogether whenever you need to go to the butcher (the hair salon or to get the newspaper), walk more. I can guarantee your health will thank you;
- **Take the stairs**: the elevator is to buildings what the car is to outside transportation; a fast, convenient but lazy way to reach your destination. As you decide to

increase your daily walking time, make a resolution to also take the stairs whenever you can;

- **Stand up**: before we became *Sapiens Sapiens*, we were *Homo Erectus* – the man that stands upright. Pay homage to your ancestors and leave your seat to pregnant women and old folks while on the bus or waiting at the post office for your number to be called. Standing straight, instead of slouching in a chair, will make your legs, butt and abs work overtime;

- **Do more chores**: here's a piece of advice that will earn you extra points with your significant other. Don't let her do all the chores. Consider doing the dishes and using the vacuum cleaner like light cardio activities. Whether you live in an apartment or a house, there's never any shortage of things to do. Mow the lawn, clean the windows, dust the shelves... Just put some music on and move with a smile!

See, cardio training doesn't have to rhyme with boredom. It's all about the mindset and finding a few routines you can stick with.

The Training Program to an Invincible Core

Alright, by now your abs should be rearing their exquisite heads if you've put into practice all we've covered thus far. Congrats! The first part of our mission is accomplished.

You can be proud of yourself but don't take your foot off the gas pedal just yet. We still got a long ways to go to build ourselves a six-pack worthy of figuring on the cover of the next Ultimate X-Men.

The Invincible Core Program

Fitness myths really are hard to die and they're waiting our every moment of inattention to hurt us. We've already talked about the "spot reduction" as well as "fat burning zone" myths.

Another misconception that the media seem especially keen on perpetuating is that of the "hundreds of reps."

The Reason Why Most Abs Programs Fail

Diet and cardio considerations aside, why do you think most people fail at getting the 6-pack of their dreams? It's not that they neglect that part... Unlike the legs or the back, that some people give as much attention to as the bum on the corner of the street, the abs do get love from most.

At the gym, the mats are seldom vacant, and you can find people killing themselves without getting as much as a second of rest. So, what gives?

No matter how many gurus would have you believe otherwise, **abs really are no different than other muscle groups**. It will do you little good to crank out hundreds of reps unless you're training for the army or preparing a Guinness Book world record.

As we talked about at the beginning of this book, we'll need to use variations on a couple of movements where the mechanical disadvantage will be going increasingly up. How can we expect to grow and become stronger if we keep repeating the exact same exercise over and over? The law of diminishing returns would soon kick in and we'd stop noticing any improvement.

Just like with high intensity cardio training, our core program will need to be short but fierce.

How We'll Handle the Issue & Ensure Success

In essence, there are 3 ways to train a muscle. You can focus your efforts on increasing its:

- Volume;
- Strength;
- Stamina.

And how exactly will you choose what factor you wish to improve? By the number of repetitions you perform.

When you go with the hundreds of reps scheme we condemned a couple of paragraphs above, you're really working on your endurance... That is, the exercises do not provide enough tension to break the muscular fibers and induce their hypertrophy; trying to build your abs this way would be like aiming to increase the size of your guns by lifting your pen until the ink inside has dried up.

To develop impressive and powerful abs, **we'll have to keep our repetitions in the 5-15 range**. The lower you go, the more you'll be working on your strength (most Olympic strength training programs are based around a 5, 3, 1 rep system.)

As for size, the general consensus is to bump that number to 6-15 reps.

Thus, we'll be staying in that range to try and get the best of both worlds. The only exception to this rule will be, as we'll discuss below, for isometric exercises; that is exercises where you'll need to maintain a given position for a certain amount of time. In that case, the number of seconds will sometimes reach higher.

3 Moves to Rise to Superhero Status

Now that we've got our rep scheme down, let's see exactly how we'll train and why we'll do it that way.

Tension in any muscle can be produced through 3 different means: by focusing on the concentric or eccentric part of a movement, or by holding a static (also called "isometric") contraction.

In the first case, which also happens to be the most common, you'll be bringing the muscle from its resting position to a fully contracted state. You'll be squeezing and shortening its fibers to the max. That's what happens to your pecs when you perform push-ups or to your biceps when you do chin-ups, for example.

When you work the eccentric part of a movement, you'll be doing the opposite; you'll be bringing the contracted muscle back to its elongated state. That's how your lats and biceps work when you learn to do a pull-up and, with the help of a chair, you get your head over the bar and concentrate on slowing down your fall. The negative part is what interests us here.

As for isometric holds, as already mentioned, you'll contract the muscle and keep it still for a given amount of time. To go back to our previous example with the pull-up, for it to be an isometric exercise, you'd have to get your head above the bar and flex your back and arms so as to keep your body in this position and not move.

To make sure our program doesn't leave any weakness in our game and is as complete as can be, we'll thus have to **make use of those 3 manners** but also be careful to **target all the different muscles we've detailed that make up the abdominals**.

And to achieve that goal, we will work towards mastering 3 difficult moves that are as complimentary as they're fun and challenging.

On top of that, you'll also get to kill two birds with one stone as those moves will make you look cooler than ever, and we both know you like to show off, don't you? C'mon, admit it!

By the time you master every progression leading to these 3 moves, your midsection will have become so strong you could take a punch in the gut from the Juggernaut and laugh about it.

Three exercises are not much, I'll give you that, but the truth is **you won't need anything else**. When you'll be struggling to finish your sets and wincing in pain, you'll remember my words and be darn happy there are no more drills following!

And without further ado, here are the meanies you'll get to know intimately in the weeks to come:

- **The Dragon Flag**: this move was one of Bruce Lee aka the Little Dragon's favorite exercises, and that's where it got its name from. The Dragon Flag can be in great part credited for Bruce's legendary abs. Abdominals so hard and powerful they could take any blow. It was, without a doubt, one of the keys that made him one of the fastest and strongest pound-for-pound fighters to ever walk this planet. With your body in a straight line from head to toes, and your weight resting on the back of your neck, you will draw half a circular arc with your feet. Or, in other words, you'll go from the vertical to the horizontal, back and forth. And as you do, you'll work the abs in all different manners, which is why the Dragon Flag is such a complete exercise (concentric phase as your feet go up; eccentric phase as they go down; isometric throughout.) This is the move to aim for if you want a crazy strong 6-pack;

- **The V-Sit**: where the Dragon Flag worked your core in its elongated state, the V-Sit will look to develop its power in the contracted position. It has no equal for building compressive power and it represents the ultimate isometric exercise. In a sense, it's what the plank dreams of becoming when it grows up; a badass move that's as humbling as it is effective! We'll go back to it in greater detail below but, for now, we'll just say that it's accomplished by pushing your hands down to lift your butt off the floor and bringing your legs straight up, gradually increasing the angle with the ground until those legs are near the vertical;

- **The Human Flag**: so far, our *rectus abdominis* will have received more than its share of work. To balance things out and target the obliques, we will introduce our most flashy move yet, the kind to make people's jaw drop in awe: the Human Flag! If your sides are a little too smooth to your taste and you wish to make them rougher and edgier, working towards achieving the Human Flag is the ideal solution. It will have them pop out like nothing! The mechanics of this move are a bit more complicated than the other two, so we'll leave the explanation for later. Just picture this: you'll be defying the laws of gravity, hanging sideways from a post like you're the solid branch of an oak, proud and strong. Sounds like fun? Hell, yeah! Here's one great exercise that will also give your arms and back a good workout.

See how useful and complimentary these 3 moves can be? If you dedicate enough time to mastering them, I can gua-ran-tee you'll secure the 6-pack you've always been craving. But before we get to them, we've got a lot of work ahead of us.

The question we ought to answer first is not so much how to perform those figures as it is **how to reach the point we're actually strong enough to do them**!

So, let's roll up our sleeves and see how we'll proceed!

Feat of Strength #01: The Exciting Road to Dragon Flag Mastery

Don't let the apparent difficulty of this move discourage you. It's like learning to paint; before you can create intricate portraits that would rival Van Gogh's most celebrated works, you first got to learn to draw a line, a shape... As your skills improve, you begin to understand how to use shading, how to make a piece more vivid or poetic.

Strength comes from practice. And in this area, nothing beats the basics. Put your pride aside and start at the very beginning; that's how you'll ensure you become a master. If your foundations are strong, nothing can go wrong!

Progression I: the Plank

The very first progression we'll address in this part is the world-renowned plank. Like I said, don't let your ego stand in the way. Don't assume it's too easy or you're too good for it. Test yourself and only pass to the next move when you've demonstrated you can actually do the required time!

By the way, this goes for every progression in this book: **don't change exercises UNTIL you've proven your worth by realizing the number or reps announced**, OK?

You'll notice, for the first few exercises, that the reps or time are pretty high, which would seem to go against everything I've been saying so far about keeping our sets short and intense... but those introductory exercises are not meant to build the size of our abs and make them more powerful. Not yet. They're part of the preparation process that will get them abs in a decent enough condition to attack the "real" work.

Take the plank, for example, you'll only be authorized to graduate to the next progression when you'll have managed to hold the position for 60 seconds. The move is easy enough... but 60 seconds is no joke!

To realize a plank:

- Get in a push-up position with your elbows locked and your back straight;
- Maintain the position.

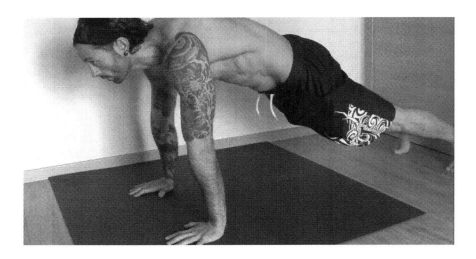

If you can't do the full minute yet, note down how long you lasted for each one of your 3 sets and try to increase the time at your next training session. Keep building until you eventually reach the target.

Progression II: the Elbow Plank
Just like the regular plank, this makes one great isometric exercise that will test the strength of your core.

Same deal: body straight in a line, but you'll be resting on your forearms instead of your hands. By shortening the "lever", you'll be bringing your body closer to the ground and changing the angle, making the exercise tougher to hold.

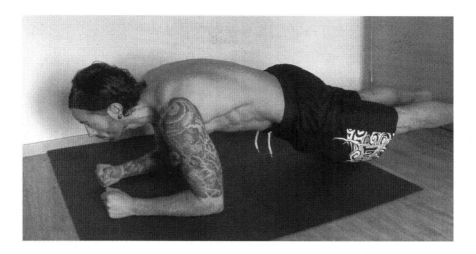

Here as well, your goal will be to hit the 60 seconds mark.

Progression III: the Inverted Plank

This is our last isometric hold before we start actually working the flag move with dynamic exercises.

In a few words, you'll be adopting a similar body position as you'll be having when you'll be doing the Dragon Flag, that is with your back to the floor in a straight line and every muscle of your body contracted.

- Lying on your back, with your arms extended behind you;
- Lift your head and your feet off the ground (don't overextend your neck or you might get hurt);
- Contract your abdominals and the muscles of your legs to ensure your body is now one big solid piece with a slight curve;
- Hold it for 60 seconds.

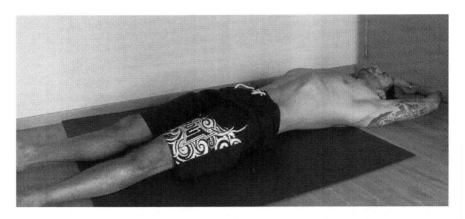

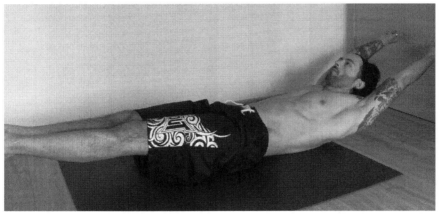

When you look at it, this move might not seem that different from a regular plank. After all, you're just keeping the same kind of position but the other way, right?

However, by inverting the move and having gravity pull down on your arms and legs, you'll notice you'll have a much harder time maintaining this posture.

Don't despair if you struggle at the beginning. Keep at it until you get the hang of it.

Progression IV: the Hand Walk

OK, you're still with me? Good! By now, your midsection should have improved noticeably. When you'll attempt the next progressions, you shouldn't feel any more cramps or pain from your abdominals overstretching a tad too much.

You've laid down the groundwork... Which means we can now finally get serious!

The exercise we'll be tackling here follows the same basic type of movement you'd be performing with an ab-wheel. You can use such a device if you already got one at home or you can refer to this no-equipment-needed variation:

- Get in a plank position, with your knees touching the ground instead of your feet;
- The goal will be to bring your head to the floor like you would if you were doing a push-up but with your arms straight;
- You will thus walk your hands forward, one after the other, until you're fully extended;
- Once you touch the ground with your forehead, come back to your starting position.

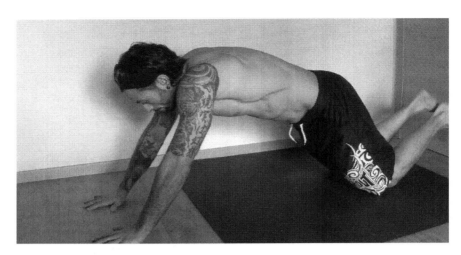

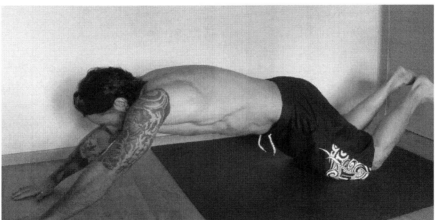

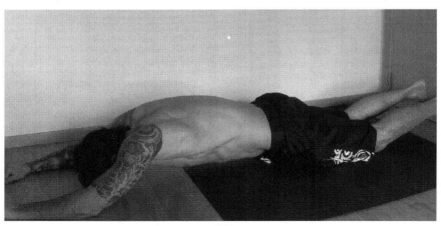

The number of reps required to move on to the next progression is 10, times 3 sets.

Progression V: the Knee Drop

Find a post or some sturdy item that's anchored in the ground for this exercise and all the others remaining in this section. Because we're finally going to work the actual flag move!

For this first variation, we will be working the eccentric portion of the Dragon Flag with the knees bent. By getting our feet closer to our core, we'll make this move much easier.

Lying down on a mat or a towel (to protect the back of your neck), with your head close to the post, almost touching it:

- Grab the post with both hands and lift your body in a candlestick, feet pointing towards the ceiling;
- Bend the knees and start lowering your legs slowly, fighting against gravity to slow down their fall;
- Once your feet touch the ground, go back up in a candlestick;
- Rinse and repeat.

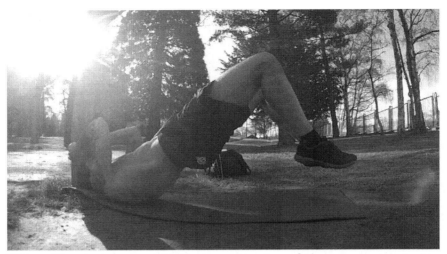

This will get you used to the mechanics of the movement. At first, when you've performed the descent, don't try to go back up keeping the dragon position locked; it will take much more strength to realize the concentric portion as simply putting the brakes on the fall.

Do keep the back straight during the eccentric part, though. Keep it in line with your thighs.

Every 10 rep of your 3 sets should last about 10 seconds, and the move should be smooth and steady. This will require quite a lot of control on your part.

Progression VI: the Straddle Drop
The movement here will be basically identical, except that you will now be extending your legs out in a straddle position instead of keeping your knees bent.

Even more so than in the previous progression, pay attention to your back the entire time. Keep it in line with your legs.

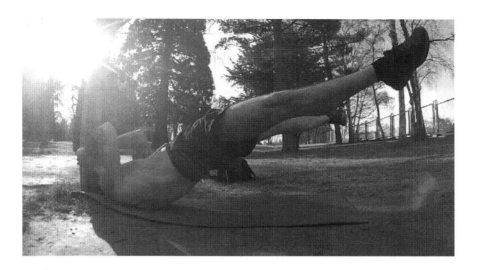

10 repetitions of 10 seconds are required to move up. Here too, perform 3 sets.

Progression VII: the Leg Drop

The last eccentric progression for the Dragon Flag will have you adopt the final position with your legs straight and closed, feet touching each other.

By bringing your legs from a straddle to a linear position, you will further accentuate the stretch and tension on your lower abdominals.

Same number of sets and repetitions required.

Progression VIII: the Half Dragon

Once you've mastered the down portion of the movement, it'll be time to add the concentric part. What comes down must eventually go up, right?

However, jumping right into the full Dragon Flag wouldn't be advised as there's still a world between the Leg Drop and this last progression. Fighting against gravity to slow down the fall of your body is much easier than fighting to have it all lift up and get to the vertical.

That's why, to begin with, you'll go for an easier variation. You'll only be doing the upper, easier half of the movement.

- Lying on the ground, holding to a post, get in a candlestick;
- With your legs straight and in line with your back, lower your legs slowly until you've reached an angle of about 45°;
- Pause for a second and return to your starting position.

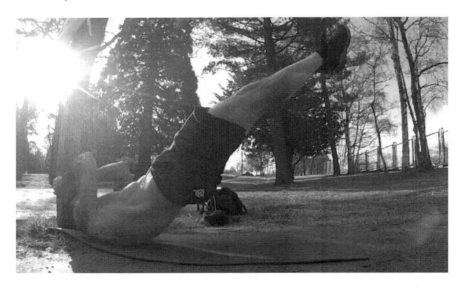

When you manage to perform 3 sets of 10 reps, you'll be ready for the real thing.

Final Progression: the Dragon Flag

This is it, the Dragon Flag! If you've been thorough thus far and really kept with the previous progressions until you could master them, this final variation should be but a formality.

This time, you'll be going through the entire range of motion, from vertical to the horizontal, and back up.

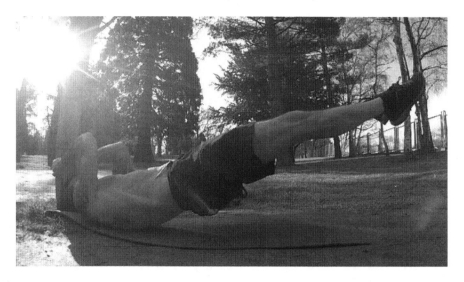

Put the Rocky theme in the background as you perform your repetitions and give your abs a workout that will make them blow up like muffins in the oven.

If you want to keep challenging them after you've taken control of this move, you can continue to make it harder by increasing the range of motion. By using an incline bench that allows you to go deeper than the horizontal, for example, you'll keep pushing their limits further and further.

You could also choose to work towards the front lever that will have you hang from a bar with your body completely parallel to the floor... but that's an entire different story.

Feat of Strength #02: How to Reach the V-Sit & Multiply Your Power Exponentially

Want to know what torture feels like but don't feel like going to Iraq? Give the V-Sit a try!

You know I'm only kidding but this exercise will truly test your spirit. Get ready to have cramps and have the wind sucked out of your lungs.

It's hard but hard work always pays off! You'll be glad you went through this ordeal when you'll have developed such compression power that you could almost ("almost" being the operative word here) haul a tank with the power of your abs.

As we did with feat #01, let's not get ahead of ourselves, though. Before we can dream about cracking nuts with our 6-pack, we first got to get it in proper condition.

Progression I: the Hanging Knee Raise

The perfect move to start working towards the V-Sit is the regular hanging knee raise. Just like the plank, it's nothing to write home about, but it's a useful exercise nonetheless to get us started on the right foot.

For this progression (and the few that follow), you'll need a pull-up bar or any object you can hang from as we'll be using our legs to provide the resistance/tension necessary to working our core.

Hanging from that bar, you will thus:

- Lift your knees up until your thighs are parallel to the floor;
- Pause for a sec;
- Bring your legs back to their resting position.

Your arms should be extended and relaxed during the entire exercise, and you should really focus on using your lower abs to have your knees move up.

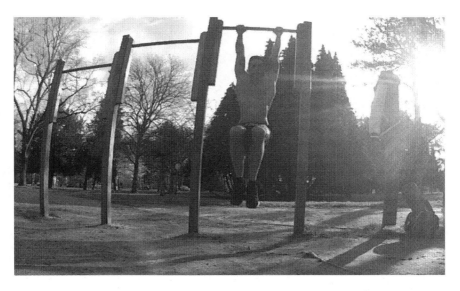

No need to deviate from our previous scheme here; 3 sets of 10 repetitions will be enough to graduate to the next variation.

Progression II: the Hanging Leg Raise

Once again, the difficulty will be upped by playing with levers and decreasing our mechanical advantage.

By keeping our legs straight instead of bending at the knees, we'll bring the weight further away from our center, which will in turn increase the torque on our abdominals.

In essence, the move will remain the same; hanging from a bar, lift your legs until they're parallel to the floor, then bring them back down in a controlled manner.

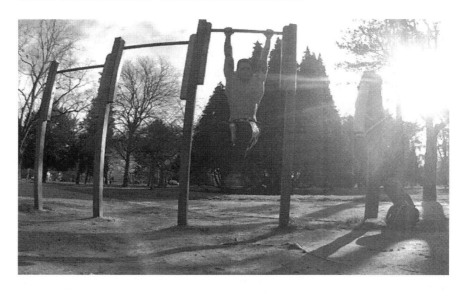

Do 3x10 reps.

Progression III: the Tuck L-Sit

OK, we've done enough raises for now; it's time to move to isometric exercises that will better mimic the mechanics of the V-Sit and which will prepare us for the later progressions.

In a way, the Tuck L-Sit can be considered to be a knee raise where you will be holding the knees up for a certain amount of time. The big difference between the two exercises, if not for the static hold, lies in the fact that the Tuck L-Sit is performed right on the floor or using parallettes.

Using your hands, you will be pushing down on the ground to depress your shoulders and raise your butt. Then, the knees will be coming up.

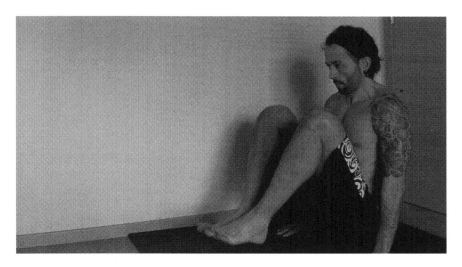

The target to reach here is 30 seconds in the air without touching your feet to the floor. As usual, do 3 sets.

Progression IV: the Tuck L-Sit with Extension
Increase the difficulty of the previous exercise by extending your legs for a brief moment.

When you're in the Tuck L-Sit position, straighten your legs, then bring them back in a tuck... That will count for 1 rep.

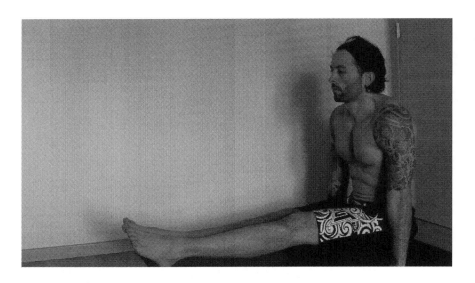

Wait until you're strong enough to perform 3 sets of 10 reps to advance to the L-Sit.

Progression V: the L-Sit

If the Dragon Flag was one of Bruce Lee's favorites, the L-Sit is definitely one of mine. It will destroy your abs and bring a smile of satisfaction to your lips.

Now, beware that your thighs and abs might cramp up at first as your muscles get used to being under such levels of tension... but the feeling eventually goes away as you toughen up and your muscular fibers turn to steel.

For the L-Sit (as for the V-Sit), even though you can execute the sets on parallettes like I said, I recommend you stick to the floor. Why? Not only because we want to be reliant on as little equipment as possible, this is the harder variation that will give you the best bang for your buck and also ensure you keep a strict form.

For the L-Sit, sitting on the ground with your legs together, you will:

- Press down with your hands to elevate your hips;
- Contract your abdominals to bring your feet in line with your pelvis;
- Hold the position with knees and elbows locked.

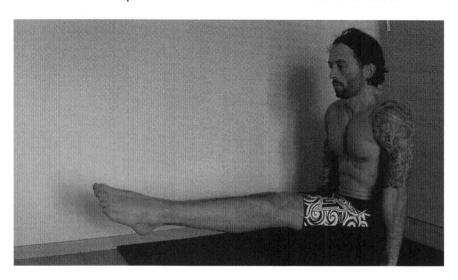

3 sets of 30 seconds will be your goal. It might take some time to build up to such numbers but if Rome wasn't built in a day, killer 6-packs never were either.

Progression VI: the Toes-to-Bar

This drill is not part of the progressions per se but rather one of the preparatory exercises. I didn't include it at the beginning for a simple reason: it requires a good deal of strength. That's why you will only start working it as you progress from L-Sit to V-Sit.

As the L-Sit becomes easier and you feel ready to "open up" the angle, add 3 sets of toes-to-bar to facilitate the transition between the two moves.

To perform toes-to-bar, hanging from a bar with your arms straight, you will:

- Pull down with your shoulder blades to stabilize the trunk;
- Tighten your midsection and, with your head going backwards, bring your feet up in an arc;
- Go up until your feet/shins touch the bar;
- Go back down while controlling the movement.

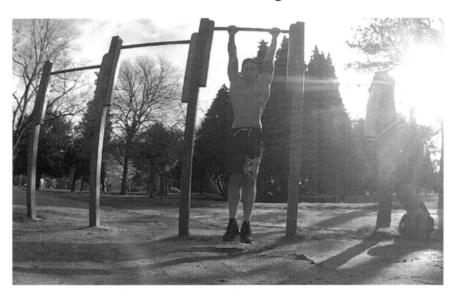

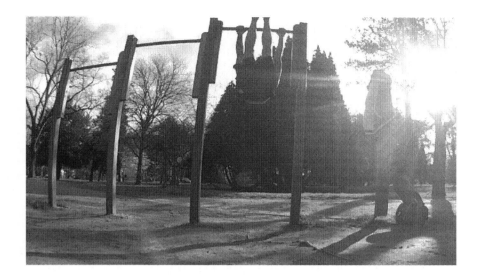

Usually, I don't have a problem with bent knees as it still gets the job done (as far as engaging the abs is concerned.) But, seeing that we will use this exercise towards building our V-Sit, which requires we keep our legs straight, we'll strive to maintain them as much in line as possible.

Flexibility might start becoming a problem at this point. If you feel it's limiting you whenever you try keeping your legs straight, add some stretching at the end of your workouts.

Build up to a dozen of reps for each set.

Final Progression: the V-Sit

The V-Sit is nothing but an L-Sit with your feet locked in a higher position than your hips... or rather an L-Sit with your legs reaching closer and closer to the vertical as if they were the hands on a watch and you were trying to turn back time.

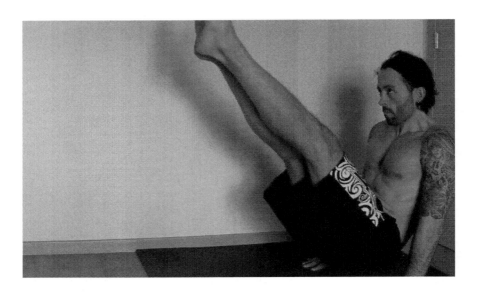

As the angle between your feet and the floor increases, you'll feel your abs getting tighter and tighter, like a foam ball you're squeezing in the palm of your hand.

This is where your compression power will shoot through the roof. Where you will develop insane levels of strength!

When you can keep the position still for about 15-20 seconds, move up a few more degrees.

Feat of Strength #03: Become Unbreakable, Become a Human Flag

Ready to claim your super powers and finally join the ranks of the elite?

If the previous moves looked cool enough and will have people take notice, this one will really bring your game to a whole new level. When you'll perform the Human Flag, it'll seem like you're defying the laws of gravity. Like you're suspended in the air like some majestic bird of prey. "Look up in the sky. It's a bird? It's a plane? No, it's Superman!"

But working towards the Human Flag will not only up your radness quotient, it will also hit your obliques and lower back hard, and guarantee a full bulletproof core.

Remember that you're only as strong as your weakest link, so we want your lumbar muscles to be as tough as your abdominals. That's why our first few exercises will focus on bringing that side up to par.

Progression I: the Superman

Before you get overly excited, reading the name of this exercise, let me warn you right away that it sounds much neater than it really is.

Compared to the final progression, it'll appear almost ridiculous... but drilling the Superman is an absolute must if you are to reach the later stages of the Human Flag.

Lying down on your belly, with your arms extended overhead:

- Lift your legs, arms and head at the same time;
- Hold the contraction for a second, really feeling it in the back and the butt;
- Return to your starting position.

If you perform the move like you should and lift your limbs high enough, it'll make you look like a rather tame version of Superman dashing through the sky, hence the name.

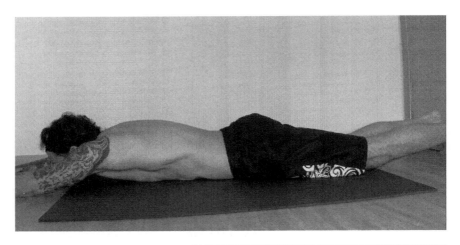

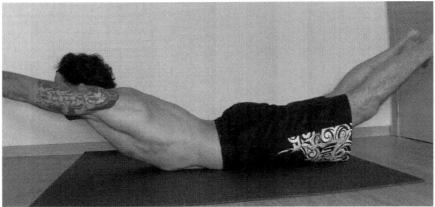

As always, pay attention to keep your arms and legs straight the whole time. Stay at it until you're strong enough to perform 3 sets of 30 reps.

Progression II: the Lower Back Raise

For the next progression, you will need someone to hold down your legs or find a way to block your feet under something as you lie down a few feet from the ground.

More lower back training here where you will be lifting your trunk up as it hangs freely in the air.

Only your legs should be in contact with the bench/table. Both your chest and abdomen will be providing the resistance to overcome. For your reps to count, you need to bring your torso all the way up so that it's now in line with your thighs.

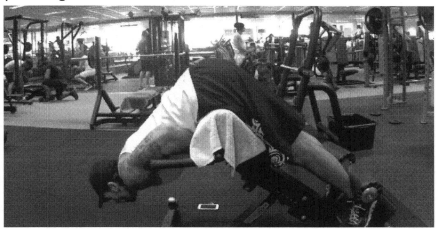

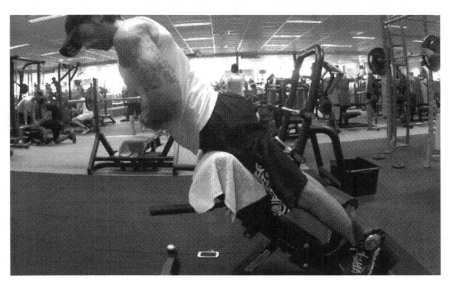

Target: 3 sets of 15 reps.

Progression III: the Side Plank

By now, your lower back should have improved enough that we can confidently turn to another weak spot that needs addressing: the obliques.

To strengthen your sides, what better way than to use the Side Plank? In the same manner that the regular Plank worked to prepare your rectus abdominis for the more advanced exercises, the Side Plank will ensure your obliques get in sufficient shape for the harder progressions to follow.

And just like the Plank, there are 2 variations to this progression, with either one hand or one forearm in contact with the floor. No time to waste, we'll go straight for the harder proposition.

Thus, you will lay sideways, your entire weight resting on your forearm and the foot on the same side. Contract the abs so the abdomen is straight in line with the rest of your body with no curve or dip in the hips.

You'll want to place your elbow right under your shoulder so your arm is perpendicular to the floor. Hold the contraction for 30 seconds before switching sides.

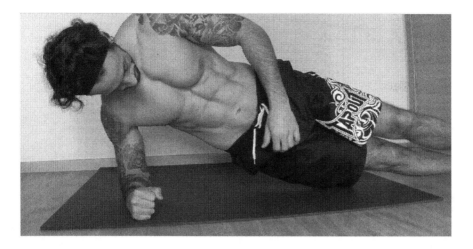

You know the drill now, 3 sets of that duration before you move to the next exercise, OK?

Progression IV: the Lying Windshield Wiper
Let's be a little more dynamic up in here, shall we? Isometric exercises like planks are very good but we need to introduce some movement to hit the abs under every angle.

To perform this progression, lie on the floor with your legs together and your arms spread cross-style to the side. Then:

- Lift your legs to the vertical;
- Using your abs to slow down their fall, bring your legs to the left side while keeping the 90° angle between your thighs and your torso constant;
- Once your feet touch the ground, go back to the vertical;
- Do the same on the right side;
- Congrats, you've done 1 rep.

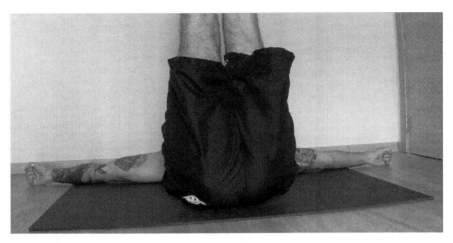

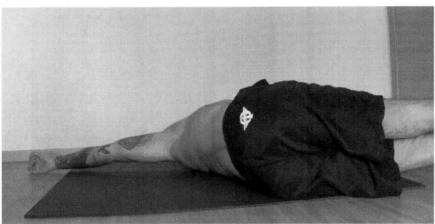

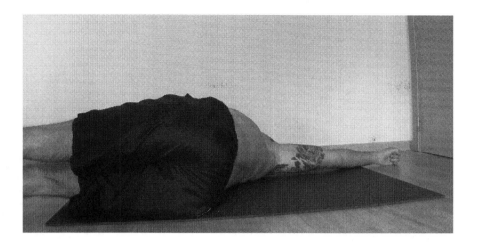

Aim for 3 sets of 15 reps.

Progression V: the Hanging Horizontal Wiper

This is basically the same move as the last one but with you hanging from a bar rather than lying down. By now, you probably know that this simple change of body position will have a substantial effect on the difficulty of the exercise.

In the previous progression, the weight of our legs was right on top of our center of gravity for a good part of the movement. Here, on the other hand, the tension will be at a maximum the entire time as your legs are extending away from start to end.

I won't go into much detail as this is basically a hanging L-Sit where you'll go from side to side with your feet, covering the whole 180°, and never once dropping the knees to get some rest.

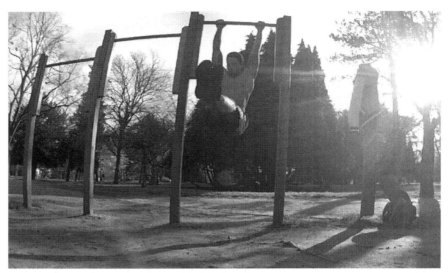

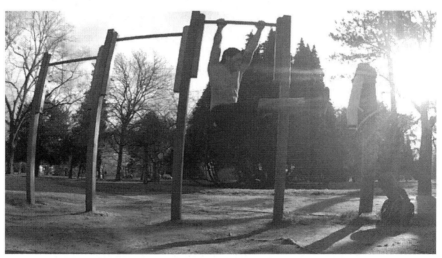

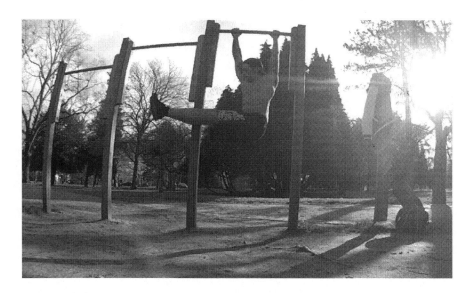

Build up to 3 sets of 10 reps on each side.

Progression VI: the Hanging Vertical Wiper

Not tough enough, you want to bump the difficulty yet another notch? Our legs are already pointing away from our center of gravity... So, how can we modify our position to make it even harder?

Answer: by bringing our feet all the way up and having our abs support even more of our bodyweight!

The starting position for this exercise will be similar to the ending position of a toes-to-bar; you will be hanging from a bar, with your arms straight, and your feet will be in contact with that bar.

Now, "all" you have left to do is to draw your half circles with your feet, like you did in the 2 previous progressions. Pay attention to keep the legs close to the body at all times and never let them fall forward. A little bending of the arms at this point is acceptable.

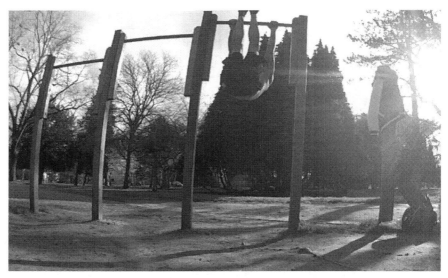

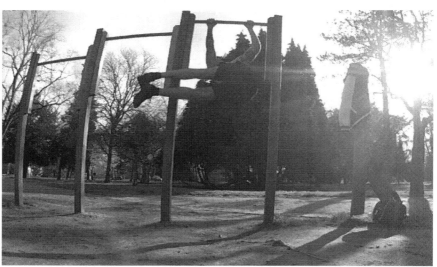

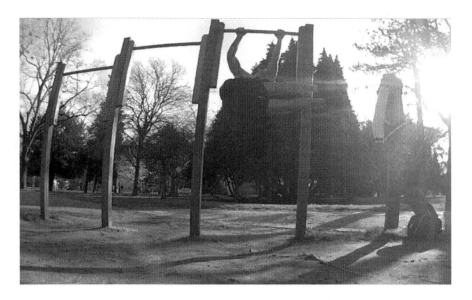

When you can manage 3 sets of 8 reps, you'll be ready to start working the actual flag.

Progression VII: the Knee Flag Drop

Before we get to it, we still need to discuss the specific mechanics of the Human Flag. You see, unlike the previous feats which were easy to grasp and intuitive, how on earth do you position yourself to get your entire body up in the air horizontally?

The trick is in producing forces which go in opposite directions. When you grab the pole, the handles or whatever you're going to do the move from, your upper hand will pull as strong as it can towards you while your lower hand will push against the support.

This play of forces will have your body rise to the side. Now, it may take some getting used to, but you'll get plenty of time to practice before you get to the last progression anyway.

For the Knee Flag Drop, you will:

- Grab the bar like I said with a greater than shoulder width grip, upper hand over the bar, lower hand under;
- Push and pull to have your torso lift up;
- Bend your legs and use the momentum to bring your knees vertically;
- Slowly return to your starting position by working the eccentric part of the movement from top to bottom.

Once again, pay attention to your arms which must remain straight the whole time.

Also, you will need a certain level of strength in the arms to be able to pull this off. That's why, if you're not training those moves already, I would strongly suggest you add push-ups and pull-ups to your training routine. This will help you progress much faster.

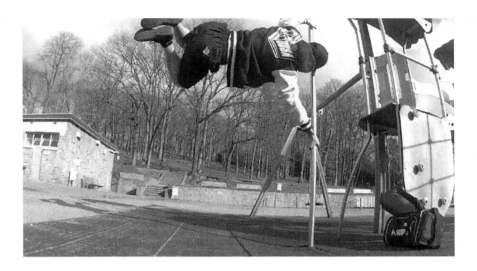

You'll want to do 3 sets of 8 reps.

Progression VIII: the Flag Drop

Same move but with the legs straight.

Start from the top and slowly lower your legs to the bottom.

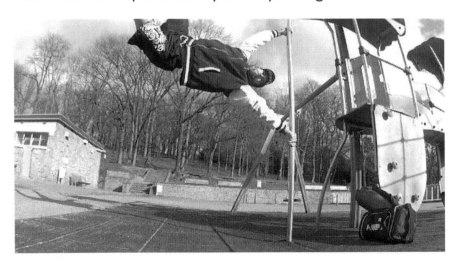

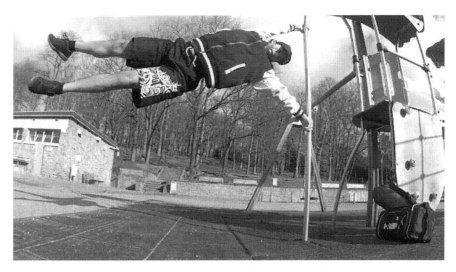

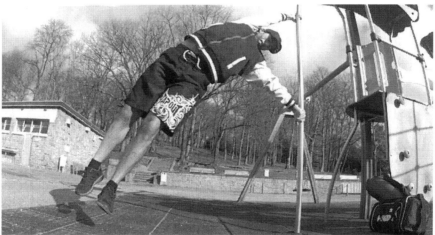

Sets and reps remain unchanged: 3x8 before you're ready for the harder variations.

Progression IX: the Knee Hold

Now and until the final progression, we will only be working in isometry. The Human Flag is essentially a static hold as you want to look like you're frozen in that eerie and impossible position.

The move isn't much different from the Knee Flag Drop. When you push and pull, and bring your knees up, instead of letting them drop to the ground you will simply – when your thighs get parallel to the floor – pause and maintain the position.

You want to be able to hold it at least 3x6 seconds before you increase the difficulty.

Progression X: the Straddle Hold
The name says it all; your legs will go into a straddle which will make the hold harder to keep but not as much as with the legs together.

The straddle (whether it's used in the planche, the flags or any other calisthenics move) may sometimes look even cooler than the progression with the legs close, but the space we put between those legs serves to improve our mechanical advantage – as we reduce the length of the lever –, thus putting less strain on the core.

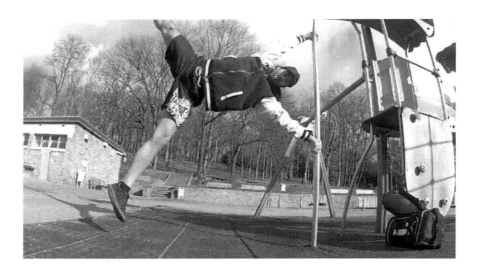

Straddle progressions are always a must before we get to the real thing.

Don't attempt the final progression until you can do your 3 sets of 6 seconds.

Final Progression: the Human Flag

You know what you have to do! You had 10 preparatory exercises to get you here, so just grab that pole, lift that butt off and show us your best Human Flag!

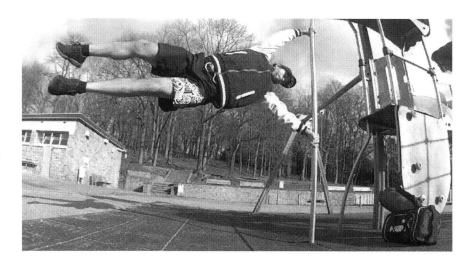

When you'll have reached this stage, your core will have become so strong and developed that, if you've followed the rest of the tips I shared with you earlier, the superhero 6-pack you coveted will have now become a reality.

This does not mean you've reached the end of the road, though. Keep pushing yourself and setting new goals. This is merely the beginning of your journey!

Putting It All Together: the Play-by-Play

OK, maybe I was a little too quick to jump to conclusion with this last paragraph and assume it was a wrap. It's one thing to read or hear about everything you need to do to reach success... but another altogether to take each one of those pieces and assemble them into a coherent program!

I know, by experience, that if we left it at that, there would be a high probability that procrastination would come up and ruin your plans of greatness.

We need to make sure we **leave you no excuse to slack off** by detailing the exact play-by-play on how your training sessions are going to unfold.

Step I: Getting It Down

Before anything else, you'll want to **write down your goals on a piece of paper**. What is it you're trying to accomplish with this program?

Whether it be to get visible abs, to be able to perform all the progressions we've seen or just to lose the gut, improve your posture and self-assurance, it's all up to you. We all have our personal reasons; there's no right or wrong answer. Only the right answer for YOU!

If you want, it could also be a good idea to take a picture of your present condition so you have a reference point for later (by the way, don't hesitate to send me your before-after pics to show me your progress.)

Once you've clarified WHY you're doing this, we'll have to determine WHEN you'll do it. Like I said, 3 sessions a week should be more than enough to ensure steady progress. In theory, you could be doing them any day of the week, when you feel like it or got enough time on your schedule... but I don't really like that approach as our levels of motivation and commitment fluctuate so much from day to day that you could end up postponing your training so much you'll miss sessions and finally give up entirely.

Fix set days (like Monday, Wednesday and Friday) and stick to them! Period.

Step II: Getting Warmed Up

Alright, now that you know exactly when you will be working out, here's how every training session will unravel.

First of all, we will need to get your muscles and your joints prepared to avoid injury. It will be especially important in the later stages when the torque on your body will be particularly intense. Unfortunately, that's one of the things people have a tendency to neglect... until something goes wrong and you pull out a muscle or worse. Then, I can assure you that you'll never train without a proper warm-up again! Don't let that be you. Do it from the get-go so you don't have to learn this lesson the hard way.

Now, to get your body loose and ready, you can do some light aerobics or perform some CrossFit moves; you can run for 5 minutes, skip rope or shadowbox if you're into fighting sports... Anything that will have your heartbeat go up and elevate your body temperature should do.

Finish up with some joint preparation. Work your shoulders, hips, wrists and neck with some rotations. All in all, this shouldn't take you more than 10 minutes... but it'll save you lots of downtime in the long run!

Step III: Working the Core

You're now all set up, ready to tackle the meat of our program. As we've seen earlier, we'll take advantage of the fact you're still fresh to work your abs and advance through the different progressions.

However, when you're just starting out, as you won't know exactly where you stand, you will want to test your skills on every one of the 3 feats.

Even if you've been working out before and built your strength to an honorable level, you will need to start at the very beginning. Don't assume you can do a progression until you've actually proven you can do it for the required time or reps!

So, on your first day, you will attempt the plank, the hanging knee raise and the Superman. If you manage the prescribed sets and numbers, congrats, you'll graduate to progression number 02 at your next training session... and so forth until you hit a wall.

Depending on your level of athleticism and sports background, you may find one of the exercises easier than the others and progress faster at first. If that's the case, don't worry, with time your lagging "parts" will catch up and you'll get stronger all across the board.

It's like when you're starting to work out; your dominant side is almost always stronger than the other and you can lift heavier weights with the muscles on that side. Eventually, as both sides improve, the gap between the two becomes thinner and thinner until one is as strong as the other.

Just make sure you work both your flags and V-Sit at every session, OK?

Which brings us to a question that probably crossed your mind as you read the previous chapters, and that is:

"How useful is it to add bodyweight exercises to our program that would target other muscle groups?"

As already stated, push-ups and pull-ups are great additional movements. Not only because they will help tremendously in acquiring the Human Flag and the V-Sit, but also because they'll make your physique even better by further developing your upper body.

So, if your question is: are those extra moves necessary or compulsory? The answer is "no."

If the question is: are they recommended? I would say "yes", without a moment's hesitation.

Step IV: Working a Sweat

You can't feel your abs anymore. You gave your core everything you got and maybe even cramped up at some point.

I applaud your dedication and salute your efforts, young warrior. But you're not done yet! Before you can go and have a shower, you've got to earn it! You've got to actually break a sweat.

Being focused on strengthening one's abdominals is laudable but it doesn't exempt you from cardio training. Remember that for those abs to show in the first place, we need to bring our calories down.

So, when you're finished with the last set of your Human Flag progressions, wrap it all up with either 10-15 minutes of HIIT or 40-60 minutes of low to moderate intensity cardio.

If you follow every one of those steps, you can't possibly fail! Your dream body is yours for the taking. The only question is: **how bad do you really want it**?

How Long Before I See Any Result?

I know, when we're just starting out, we're often overly eager. We feel that fire burning inside. But this eagerness can be a double-edged sword. On one hand, we have motivation for days; on the other, we can be equally impatient.

We want results and we want them for yesterday! So, how long can you expect to wait before you witness any change in your appearance?

It's kind of hard to give any timeframe. It's like asking how long it would take you to go to Vegas. Will you go by plane, by car or on foot? Will you be making frequent stops or will you cover the entire distance at once? As if things weren't complicated enough, some people are faster than others... and we're not all launching from the same starting point!

Your results will obviously depend on your diligence and levels of commitment, but also on your diet and whether or not you'll be doing cardio work. It will also be reliant on your starting shape and the goals you set out to achieve.

But as a rule of thumb, I would say that if you look more like a regular Joe than a sumo, **anywhere from 6 to 12 weeks** should do the trick.

This is no "get abs while you sleep" program... but I can assure you that THIS works and, as long as you don't quit, you're destined to make it.

Conclusion: from Dream to Reality

Dreams are only as good as they propel you into action. If they don't fuel your inner fire and get you to move your butt, they're really no better than cheap B movies you watch at night when you're bored. They pass time but they'll never change your life!

Securing a superhero six-pack is within your reach. You can start acting today and have your vision become reality. Or you can leave that image of a superior You in fantasy land where it'll slowly wither and die. Like all those other dreams you never acted upon.

The choice is ultimately yours. No matter how much I'd love to be able to reach through this book with a virtual hand, grab you by the shoulders and shake you stupid when you need it the most... I'm afraid my job stops here.

I've shared everything you needed to know to slim down, develop a monster core and regain both your health and self-confidence. **The theory now has to lead to practice!**

Referring back to the information we covered:

- Write down your goals;
- Choose which type of diet you'll be following;
- Determine on which days of the week you'll be training;

- For each session, warm yourself up, work your abs using the right progressions, and finish off with some cardio.

How easier could it really get?

Now, go and make a difference in your life. Wake up and get busy. **You've been dreaming long enough**!

Want to Reach Your Full Potential?

If you feel like getting serious and investing in yourself, check out the "**Real Life Superman**" series; my progressive method to become the very best version of yourself you can be:

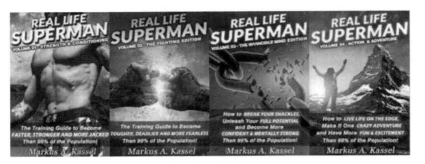

Volume I: the Strength & Conditioning Edition – Build Muscle, Increase Your Stamina and Become a True War Machine;

Volume II: the Fighting Edition – Learn How to Become Tougher, Deadlier and More Fearless;

Volume III: the Invincible Mind Edition – Free Your Mind from Its Shackles and Unleash Your Full Potential;

Volume IV: the Action & Adventure Edition – Seize Every Opportunity and Make an Adventure of Your Life.

Let's Keep In Touch

Now that this book comes to an end, I'd like to extend a hand to you. I feel like we're somehow connected now. I hope that the content of this guide resonated with you and your past experiences, that you could identify with my journey, my ambitions and setbacks. If that's the case, no matter where you are in life today, we're kindred spirits with yet a lot to share!

That's why I'd like to keep in touch; so we can continue to progress together. We've both embarked on a road that knows no end, a road to perfection that can sometimes get very lonely when no one else around you can relate. We can offer each other that support. We can help each other become better!

Whether you have a question to ask, a comment or suggestion you'd like to make, or if you simply want to tell me about your goals and the progress you've already made, you can reach me:

Via my site: http://reallifesuperman.com

Or my email address: markus@reallifesuperman.com

It'll be my pleasure to help!

Speaking of help, if you have 2 minutes to spare, I'd like to ask for yours. I need your feedback to find out if I'm on the right track. If you could do me a favor and drop a word or two about this book on Amazon, it would mean the world to me!

I thank you in advance and I'll see you soon, my friend.

About the Author

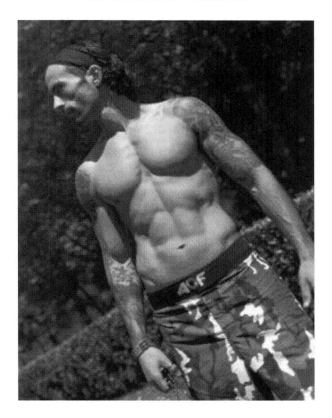

A black belt in Karate, ring-tested kickboxer who also holds a university degree in Psychology, I have to admit I know a thing or two about kicking butt and imposing my will on my foes. However, the real adversary I've always been looking to vanquish — whether in CrossFit competitions, in a race or a fight — has never been anyone else but me.

I believe in the Latin phrase *mens sana in corpore sano* and try to honor that spirit every chance I get by looking for new, more efficient ways to improve myself and reach the next level. Through my trials and errors, I've accumulated a vast wealth of knowledge. Not only on the **quickest means to attain one's physical peak** but also on what it takes to **toughen up mentally and develop a sharp, indestructible mind**.

In this series of books, I intend to share with you everything I've learned in close to 20 years of studying and perfecting my training. It is the next natural step for me: to put into words all that baggage made of sensations, hard-earned habits and unspoken truths; to extract its very essence without holding anything back. And by so doing, not only will I get better, you will as well!

Some of the facts I'll lay out will surprise you, others may come as a shock, but rest assured that they represent the **fastest shortcut to success**. So, if you're ready for the change of a lifetime, let's get started and discover the Superhero who had been hiding inside you all along!

Sincerely,

Markus

Made in the USA
Middletown, DE
06 March 2017